SUPERB WEIGHT LOSS COOKBOOK FOR BEGINNERS 2024

Effortless Meals to Kick start Your Weight Loss Journey

MARY M. VANISH

Disclaimer

The information provided in "Superb Weight Loss Cookbook for Beginners 2024" is intended for educational and informational purposes only and is not intended as medical advice. Always consult your physician or other qualified health provider with any questions you may have regarding a medical condition or before beginning any diet or exercise program. The author and publisher are not responsible for any adverse effects or consequences resulting from the use of any recipes, suggestions, or procedures described in this book.

Every effort has been made to ensure that the information in this book is accurate and complete as of the date of publication. However, the author and publisher make no representations or warranties regarding the completeness, accuracy, or reliability of the information contained herein. Any reliance on the material in this book is at your own risk.

Individual results from the use of recipes and suggestions in this book may vary and are dependent on many factors including but not limited to individual body constitution, health conditions, and adherence to the suggestions provided.

By using this book, you agree to indemnify, defend, and hold harmless the author and publisher from any and all claims, liability, damages, and/or costs arising from your use of the information provided herein.

Mary M. Vanish

ABOUT THE AUTHOR

Mary M. Vanish is a passionate advocate for healthy living and nutritious cooking. With a lifelong dedication to promoting wellness through wholesome, balanced meals, Mary has become a respected voice in the culinary world. Her journey began in her grandmother's kitchen, where she first discovered the joys of preparing fresh, home-cooked meals. This early experience ignited a lifelong passion for cooking that has only grown stronger over the years.

Mary pursued her formal education in nutrition and culinary arts, earning a degree that provided a solid foundation for her career. She has worked as a professional chef, nutritionist, and culinary educator, always striving to combine her love of food with her commitment to health. Her culinary philosophy is simple: healthy eating should be delicious, accessible, and enjoyable for everyone.

In addition to her professional work, Mary has been a tireless advocate for community health initiatives. She has conducted numerous workshops and cooking classes, helping people from all walks of life understand the importance of nutritious eating and how to prepare healthy meals at home. Her approachable teaching style and genuine enthusiasm for healthy cooking have inspired countless individuals to take charge of their health through better nutrition.

Mary's dedication to healthy cooking extends beyond the kitchen. She is an active supporter of local farmers' markets and sustainable agriculture, believing that fresh, locally-sourced ingredients are key to both great flavor and good health. She also collaborates with schools and community organizations to promote nutrition education and healthy eating habits among children and families.

"Superb Weight Loss Cookbook for Beginners 2024" is a testament to Mary's expertise and her unwavering commitment to helping others lead healthier lives. In this book, she shares her knowledge, tips, and delicious recipes designed to support weight loss and overall wellness. Each recipe reflects her belief that healthy food should not only nourish the body but also delight the senses.

When she's not in the kitchen, Mary enjoys spending time with her family, exploring nature, and experimenting with new recipes. She lives by the mantra that every meal is an opportunity to celebrate life and nourish the body. Through her writing, Mary hopes to inspire others to embrace the joys of healthy eating and discover the transformative power of nutritious, home-cooked meals.

Table of Contents

INTRODUCTION

Welcome to "Superb Weight Loss Cookbook for Beginners 2024"! This book is your gateway to a healthier, more vibrant life, filled with delicious meals that support your weight loss journey. Whether you're new to cooking or just beginning to explore healthy eating, this cookbook is designed to make your path to wellness both enjoyable and accessible.

In today's fast-paced world, maintaining a healthy diet can often feel overwhelming. The abundance of conflicting information about what to eat and the allure of convenient, yet unhealthy, food choices make it challenging to stay on track. That's where this book comes in. With clear guidance, practical tips, and a collection of tasty, nutrient-rich recipes, you'll discover that eating well and losing weight can be both simple and satisfying.

The recipes in this cookbook are thoughtfully crafted to balance taste and nutrition. Each dish is designed to nourish your body while helping you achieve and maintain a healthy weight. From hearty breakfasts that jumpstart your day to comforting dinners that bring your evenings to a satisfying close, you'll find a variety of meals that cater to your taste buds and nutritional needs.

But this book is more than just a collection of recipes. It's a comprehensive guide to healthy living. You'll find chapters dedicated to understanding the basics of nutrition, meal planning, and smart grocery shopping. These sections provide the foundational knowledge you need to make informed choices and create a sustainable eating plan that works for you.

Throughout these pages, you'll also find practical tips and strategies for overcoming common obstacles to healthy eating. Learn how to navigate social events, manage cravings, and maintain motivation. Discover the benefits of mindful eating and how to develop a positive relationship with food. This holistic approach ensures that you're not only losing weight but also building habits that promote long-term health and wellness.

What sets this cookbook apart is its emphasis on simplicity and accessibility. Each recipe includes clear instructions, making it easy for beginners to follow along. The ingredients are readily available, and the preparation methods are straightforward, ensuring that you can create delicious, healthy meals without spending hours in the kitchen.

As you embark on this journey, remember that healthy eating is not about deprivation or rigid dieting. It's about finding joy in nourishing your body and discovering flavors that excite you. It's about making small, sustainable changes that lead to big results. And most importantly, it's about taking care of yourself and celebrating every step you take towards a healthier you.

Thank you for choosing "Superb Weight Loss Cookbook for Beginners 2024." I'm thrilled to join you on this journey and can't wait to see the positive changes it brings to your life. Here's to a healthier, happier you!

Warmest regards,

CHAPTER

BREAKFAST BOOSTERS

1. Green Smoothie Bowl

A Nutritious Start to Your Day

Serving Size: 1 bowl
Prep Time: 10 minutes
Cooking Time: None

Nutrition Information (per serving):

- Calories: 300
- Protein: 10g
- Carbohydrates: 40g
- Dietary Fiber: 8g
- Sugars: 20g
- Fat: 10g
- Saturated Fat: 2g
- Vitamin A: 150% DV
- Vitamin C: 100% DV
- Calcium: 15% DV
- Iron: 20% DV

Ingredients:

- 1 banana, sliced and frozen
- 1/2 cup frozen spinach
- 1/2 cup frozen mango chunks
- 1/2 avocado
- 1/2 cup unsweetened almond milk (or any preferred milk)
- 1 tablespoon chia seeds
- 1 tablespoon almond butter (optional)
- 1 teaspoon honey or maple syrup (optional)
- Toppings: fresh berries, granola, sliced banana, chia seeds, coconut flakes, or nuts

Directions:

1. **Blend the Base:** In a high-speed blender, combine the frozen banana, frozen spinach, frozen mango chunks, avocado, and almond milk. Blend until smooth and creamy. If the mixture is too thick, add a bit more almond milk to reach your desired consistency.
2. **Sweeten to Taste:** Add the chia seeds and, if desired, the almond butter and honey or maple syrup. Blend again until everything is well incorporated.
3. **Serve:** Pour the smoothie into a bowl.
4. **Add Toppings:** Top your smoothie bowl with your favorite toppings. Popular choices include

fresh berries, granola, sliced banana, chia seeds, coconut flakes, and nuts. These add texture, flavor, and additional nutrients.

5. **Enjoy Immediately:** Green smoothie bowls are best enjoyed fresh. Grab a spoon and dig in!

Tips for a Perfect Smoothie Bowl:

- **Frozen Ingredients:** Using frozen fruits and vegetables creates a thicker, creamier smoothie bowl.
- **Customize:** Feel free to customize your smoothie bowl by adding different fruits, greens, or superfood powders.
- **Balanced Nutrition:** Adding a source of healthy fat, like avocado or nut butter, helps balance the natural sugars from the fruit and keeps you full longer.

2. Protein-Packed Veggie Omelette

Serving Size

Servings: 1

Cooking Time

Prep Time: 10 minutes
Cooking Time: 10 minutes

Nutrition Information (per serving)

- Calories: 250
- Protein: 20g
- Carbohydrates: 8g
- Fat: 16g
- Fiber: 2g

Ingredients

- 3 large eggs (or 2 eggs and 2 egg whites for a lower fat option)
- 1/4 cup diced bell pepper (any color)
- 1/4 cup diced tomatoes
- 1/4 cup spinach leaves, chopped
- 1/4 cup mushrooms, sliced
- 1/4 cup shredded low-fat cheese (optional)
- 1/4 cup cooked quinoa or black beans (optional for extra protein)
- 1 tablespoon olive oil or cooking spray
- Salt and pepper to taste
- Fresh herbs (optional, for garnish)

Directions

1. **Prepare the Ingredients:**
   - Dice the bell pepper and tomatoes.

- Chop the spinach leaves.
- Slice the mushrooms.
- If using quinoa or black beans, ensure they are cooked and ready to use.

2. **Beat the Eggs:**
   - In a bowl, beat the eggs until well mixed. Season with a pinch of salt and pepper.

3. **Cook the Vegetables:**
   - In a non-stick skillet, heat the olive oil over medium heat.
   - Add the bell pepper, tomatoes, spinach, and mushrooms to the skillet.
   - Sauté for 2-3 minutes until the vegetables are tender and the spinach is wilted.

4. **Add the Eggs:**
   - Pour the beaten eggs over the sautéed vegetables, spreading them evenly in the skillet.
   - Allow the eggs to cook undisturbed for a minute until the edges start to set.

5. **Add Cheese and Protein (Optional):**
   - Sprinkle the shredded cheese evenly over the omelette if using.
   - Add the cooked quinoa or black beans for an extra protein boost.

6. **Cook Until Set:**
   - Using a spatula, gently lift the edges of the omelette to let any uncooked egg flow underneath.

- Cook for another 2-3 minutes until the eggs are fully set but still slightly moist on top.
7. **Fold and Serve:**
   - Carefully fold the omelette in half and slide it onto a plate.
   - Garnish with fresh herbs if desired.

3. Overnight Chia Pudding

Serving Size: 2
Prep Time: 10 minutes
Chill Time: 4 hours (or overnight)
Total Time: 4 hours 10 minutes

Nutritional Information (per serving):

- Calories: 180
- Protein: 6g
- Carbohydrates: 24g
- Fiber: 10g
- Sugars: 8g
- Fat: 8g
- Saturated Fat: 2g

Ingredients:

- 1/4 cup chia seeds

- 1 cup unsweetened almond milk (or any milk of your choice)
- 1 tablespoon honey or maple syrup (optional for sweetness)
- 1/2 teaspoon vanilla extract
- Fresh fruits, nuts, and seeds for topping (optional)

Directions:

1. **Mix Ingredients:**
   - In a medium-sized bowl, combine the chia seeds, almond milk, honey (if using), and vanilla extract.
   - Stir the mixture thoroughly to ensure that the chia seeds are evenly distributed and not clumping together.
2. **Chill:**
   - Cover the bowl with plastic wrap or transfer the mixture to an airtight container.
   - Place it in the refrigerator for at least 4 hours, but preferably overnight. This allows the chia seeds to absorb the liquid and form a pudding-like consistency.
3. **Stir Again:**
   - After the first 30 minutes of chilling, give the mixture a good stir to prevent the chia seeds from settling at the

bottom. Return it to the refrigerator to continue setting.

4. **Serve:**
   - Once the chia pudding has thickened, give it one final stir.
   - Divide the pudding into two serving bowls.

5. **Add Toppings:**
   - Top with your favorite fresh fruits, nuts, and seeds for added flavor, texture, and nutrition. Some popular choices include sliced bananas, berries, almonds, and pumpkin seeds.

6. **Enjoy:**
   - Serve immediately or keep it refrigerated for up to 3 days.

Benefits of Chia Pudding

Chia pudding is not only delicious but also packed with nutrients. Chia seeds are a great source of omega-3 fatty acids, fiber, protein, and various essential minerals. This easy-to-make breakfast helps you feel full and energized throughout the morning, making it an excellent choice for weight loss and overall health.

Customization Tips

Feel free to customize your chia pudding by adding different flavors and ingredients. You can mix in cocoa powder for a chocolate version, use coconut milk for a tropical twist, or sweeten it with mashed fruits instead of honey. The possibilities are endless!

4. Avocado Toast with Poached Egg

Serving Size: 1
Prep Time: 10 minutes
Cooking Time: 5 minutes

Nutrition Information (per serving):

- Calories: 300
- Protein: 12g
- Carbohydrates: 20g
- Fat: 20g
- Fiber: 8g
- Sugar: 2g

Ingredients:

- 1 slice whole-grain bread
- 1/2 ripe avocado
- 1 large egg
- 1 tsp white vinegar
- Salt and pepper to taste
- Optional toppings: cherry tomatoes, red pepper flakes, chives, or a squeeze of lemon juice

Directions:

1. **Toast the Bread:** Begin by toasting the whole-grain bread slice to your desired level of crispiness.
2. **Prepare the Avocado:** While the bread is toasting, cut the avocado in half, remove the pit, and scoop the flesh into a small bowl. Mash the avocado with a fork until it reaches a creamy consistency. Add a pinch of salt and pepper for flavor.
3. **Poach the Egg:** Fill a small saucepan with water and bring it to a gentle simmer. Add the white vinegar to the water. Crack the egg into a small bowl or ramekin. Create a gentle whirlpool in the simmering water with a spoon and carefully slide the egg into the center of the whirlpool. Poach the egg for about 3-4 minutes, until the white is set but the yolk is still runny. Remove the egg with a slotted spoon and gently pat it dry with a paper towel.
4. **Assemble the Toast:** Spread the mashed avocado evenly over the toasted bread. Place the poached egg on top of the avocado.
5. **Season and Serve:** Sprinkle with additional salt and pepper to taste. Add optional toppings like cherry tomatoes, red pepper flakes, chives, or a squeeze of lemon juice for extra flavor. Serve immediately.

5. Quinoa Breakfast Bowl

Serving Size: 1 bowl
Prep Time: 10 minutes
Cooking Time: 15 minutes

Nutrition Information (Per Serving)

- **Calories:** 350
- **Protein:** 12g
- **Carbohydrates:** 55g
- **Fiber:** 7g
- **Fat:** 10g
- **Sugar:** 10g

Ingredients

- 1/2 cup quinoa, rinsed
- 1 cup water or milk (dairy or plant-based)
- 1/2 cup mixed berries (blueberries, strawberries, raspberries)
- 1 small banana, sliced
- 1 tbsp chia seeds
- 1 tbsp almond butter or peanut butter
- 1 tsp honey or maple syrup (optional)
- A pinch of cinnamon

- Fresh mint leaves for garnish (optional)

Directions

1. **Cook the Quinoa:**
   - In a medium saucepan, combine the rinsed quinoa and water (or milk). Bring to a boil over medium-high heat.
   - Once boiling, reduce the heat to low, cover, and let it simmer for about 15 minutes or until the quinoa has absorbed all the liquid and is tender. Remove from heat and let it sit for 5 minutes, then fluff with a fork.
2. **Assemble the Bowl:**
   - Transfer the cooked quinoa to a serving bowl.
   - Arrange the mixed berries and sliced banana on top of the quinoa.
3. **Add Toppings:**
   - Sprinkle the chia seeds over the fruits.
   - Drizzle the almond butter or peanut butter over the top.
   - If desired, add a drizzle of honey or maple syrup for extra sweetness.
4. **Garnish and Serve:**
   - Add a pinch of cinnamon for extra flavor.

- Garnish with fresh mint leaves, if using.
5. **Enjoy:**
   - Mix everything together before eating, or savor each layer individually. Enjoy your delicious and nutritious Quinoa Breakfast Bowl!

Tips for Customization

- **Fruit Variations:** Swap out the berries and banana for your favorite fruits like apples, pears, or mango.
- **Protein Boost:** Add a scoop of Greek yogurt or a sprinkle of nuts and seeds for an extra protein boost.
- **Flavor Twist:** Try different nut butters like cashew or sunflower seed butter, and experiment with spices like nutmeg or vanilla extract.

6. Cottage Cheese and Fruit Parfait

Servings: 2
Prep Time: 10 minutes
Cooking Time: None

Nutrition Information (per serving):

- Calories: 200
- Protein: 15g
- Carbohydrates: 25g
- Fat: 5g
- Fiber: 3g
- Sugar: 18g

Ingredients:

- 1 cup low-fat cottage cheese
- 1/2 cup strawberries, sliced
- 1/2 cup blueberries
- 1/2 cup kiwi, diced
- 1/2 cup granola (preferably low-sugar)
- 2 tbsp honey or agave syrup (optional)
- Fresh mint leaves for garnish (optional)

Directions:

1. **Prepare the Ingredients:** Wash and slice the strawberries, dice the kiwi, and wash the blueberries. Set aside.
2. **Layer the Parfait:** In two medium-sized glasses or bowls, start by adding 1/4 cup of cottage cheese to the bottom of each.
3. **Add Fruit Layers:** Add a layer of strawberries, followed by a layer of blueberries, and then a layer of kiwi. Divide the fruit evenly between the two servings.

4. **Top with Cottage Cheese:** Add another 1/4 cup of cottage cheese on top of the fruit layers in each glass.
5. **Finish with Granola:** Sprinkle 1/4 cup of granola over the top of each parfait for a crunchy texture.
6. **Optional Sweetener:** Drizzle 1 tablespoon of honey or agave syrup over each parfait for added sweetness, if desired.
7. **Garnish and Serve:** Garnish with fresh mint leaves for a touch of color and freshness. Serve immediately and enjoy!

CHAPTER 2
LIGHT AND SATISFYING LUNCHES

1. Quinoa and Avocado Salad

Serving Size, Cooking Time, and Prep Time

- **Serving Size:** 4
- **Cooking Time:** 15 minutes
- **Prep Time:** 15 minutes

Nutrition Information (per serving)

- **Calories:** 350
- **Protein:** 8g
- **Fat:** 20g
- **Carbohydrates:** 35g
- **Fiber:** 10g
- **Sugars:** 3g

Ingredients

- 1 cup quinoa
- 2 cups water
- 1 large avocado, diced
- 1 cup cherry tomatoes, halved
- 1/2 cup red onion, finely chopped
- 1 cucumber, diced
- 1/4 cup fresh cilantro, chopped
- 1/4 cup olive oil
- Juice of 1 lime
- Salt and pepper to taste

Directions

1. **Cook the Quinoa:**
   - Rinse quinoa under cold water.
   - In a medium pot, bring 2 cups of water to a boil.
   - Add quinoa, reduce heat to low, cover, and simmer for about 15 minutes, or until the water is absorbed and the quinoa is tender.
   - Remove from heat and let it sit, covered, for 5 minutes. Fluff with a fork and let it cool.
2. **Prepare the Vegetables:**
   - While the quinoa is cooking, dice the avocado, halve the cherry tomatoes, finely chop the red onion, and dice the cucumber.
   - Chop the fresh cilantro.
3. **Make the Dressing:**

- In a small bowl, whisk together the olive oil, lime juice, salt, and pepper.
4. **Assemble the Salad:**
   - In a large bowl, combine the cooked and cooled quinoa, diced avocado, cherry tomatoes, red onion, cucumber, and cilantro.
   - Pour the dressing over the salad and toss gently to combine, ensuring all ingredients are evenly coated.
5. **Serve:**
   - Divide the salad among four plates or bowls.
   - Serve immediately or refrigerate for up to 2 hours to allow the flavors to meld.

Tips for Success

- For added flavor, consider toasting the quinoa in a dry pan for a few minutes before cooking.
- Feel free to customize the salad by adding other veggies like bell peppers or leafy greens.
- This salad pairs well with grilled chicken or fish for a more substantial meal.

2. Chicken and Veggie Lettuce Wraps

Serving Size: 4 wraps
Prep Time: 15 minutes
Cooking Time: 15 minutes

Nutrition Information (per serving):

- Calories: 220
- Protein: 22g
- Carbohydrates: 15g
- Fiber: 5g
- Fat: 8g

Ingredients:

- 1 lb ground chicken
- 1 tbsp olive oil
- 1 red bell pepper, diced
- 1 cup carrots, shredded
- 1 cup mushrooms, finely chopped
- 1/2 cup water chestnuts, chopped
- 2 cloves garlic, minced
- 2 tbsp soy sauce (low sodium)
- 1 tbsp hoisin sauce
- 1 tsp rice vinegar
- 1 head of butter or iceberg lettuce, leaves separated
- 1/4 cup green onions, sliced
- 1/4 cup cilantro, chopped
- Salt and pepper to taste

Directions:

1. **Prepare the Ingredients:** Wash and dry the lettuce leaves. Set aside. Dice the red bell pepper, shred the carrots, and finely chop the mushrooms and water chestnuts.
2. **Cook the Chicken:** In a large skillet, heat olive oil over medium heat. Add ground chicken and cook until browned, breaking it apart with a spoon, about 5-7 minutes. Season with salt and pepper.
3. **Add the Vegetables:** Add garlic, red bell pepper, carrots, mushrooms, and water chestnuts to the skillet. Cook until the vegetables are tender, about 5 minutes.
4. **Add the Sauces:** Stir in soy sauce, hoisin sauce, and rice vinegar. Cook for an additional 2 minutes, allowing the flavors to combine.
5. **Assemble the Wraps:** Remove the skillet from heat. Spoon the chicken and vegetable mixture onto the center of each lettuce leaf.
6. **Garnish and Serve:** Sprinkle with sliced green onions and chopped cilantro. Fold the lettuce leaf around the filling like a wrap and serve immediately.

Tips for Making Perfect Lettuce Wraps:

- **Choosing Lettuce:** Butter lettuce and iceberg lettuce work best for wraps due to their sturdy leaves.
- **Preparation:** Ensure the lettuce leaves are dry to prevent them from becoming soggy.
- **Variations:** Feel free to add other vegetables or use ground turkey instead of chicken for a different flavor profile.

3. Mediterranean Chickpea Salad

Prep Time: 15 minutes
Cooking Time: 0 minutes
Serving Size: 4

Nutrition Information (per serving):

- Calories: 240
- Protein: 8g
- Carbohydrates: 30g
- Dietary Fiber: 7g
- Sugars: 4g
- Fat: 10g
- Saturated Fat: 1.5g
- Sodium: 400mg

Ingredients:

- 1 can (15 oz) chickpeas, drained and rinsed
- 1 cup cherry tomatoes, halved
- 1 cucumber, diced
- 1/2 red onion, finely chopped
- 1/4 cup Kalamata olives, pitted and sliced
- 1/4 cup crumbled feta cheese
- 2 tbsp fresh parsley, chopped
- 2 tbsp extra-virgin olive oil
- 1 tbsp red wine vinegar
- 1 clove garlic, minced
- 1 tsp dried oregano
- Salt and pepper to taste

Directions:

1. **Prepare the Vegetables:** Start by chopping the cherry tomatoes, cucumber, red onion, and Kalamata olives. Make sure all the vegetables are bite-sized for easy eating.
2. **Mix the Salad:** In a large bowl, combine the drained chickpeas, cherry tomatoes, cucumber, red onion, and Kalamata olives. Toss gently to mix all the ingredients evenly.
3. **Add Cheese and Herbs:** Sprinkle the crumbled feta cheese and chopped parsley over the salad mixture.
4. **Prepare the Dressing:** In a small bowl, whisk together the extra-virgin olive oil, red wine vinegar, minced garlic, dried oregano, salt, and pepper until well combined.

5. **Dress the Salad:** Pour the dressing over the salad and toss gently to ensure all the ingredients are well coated with the dressing.
6. **Serve:** Divide the salad into four servings and enjoy immediately or refrigerate for up to two days. This salad is perfect as a light lunch or as a side dish to complement grilled meats or fish.

Tips:

- For extra flavor, you can add a squeeze of fresh lemon juice to the dressing.
- To make this salad a more substantial meal, consider adding some grilled chicken or shrimp on top.

4. Grilled Shrimp and Veggie Skewers

Serving Size: 4
Prep Time: 20 minutes
Cooking Time: 10 minutes

Nutrition Information (per serving):

- Calories: 220
- Protein: 25g
- Carbohydrates: 10g

- Fat: 10g
- Fiber: 3g
- Sodium: 600mg

Ingredients:

- 1 lb large shrimp, peeled and deveined
- 1 red bell pepper, cut into chunks
- 1 yellow bell pepper, cut into chunks
- 1 zucchini, sliced into thick rounds
- 1 red onion, cut into chunks
- 1 cup cherry tomatoes
- 3 tbsp olive oil
- 2 tbsp lemon juice
- 3 cloves garlic, minced
- 1 tsp paprika
- 1 tsp dried oregano
- Salt and pepper to taste
- Skewers (if using wooden skewers, soak in water for at least 30 minutes)

Directions:

1. **Prepare the Marinade:**
   - In a bowl, combine olive oil, lemon juice, minced garlic, paprika, dried oregano, salt, and pepper. Mix well to form a marinade.
2. **Marinate the Shrimp:**
   - Add the shrimp to the marinade and toss to coat. Let marinate for at least

15 minutes while you prepare the vegetables.

3. **Prepare the Vegetables:**
   - In a separate bowl, combine the bell peppers, zucchini, red onion, and cherry tomatoes. Drizzle with a little olive oil, and season with salt and pepper. Toss to coat.

4. **Assemble the Skewers:**
   - Thread the shrimp and vegetables onto the skewers, alternating between shrimp, bell peppers, zucchini, red onion, and cherry tomatoes. Repeat until all ingredients are used.

5. **Preheat the Grill:**
   - Preheat your grill to medium-high heat.

6. **Grill the Skewers:**
   - Place the skewers on the preheated grill. Cook for 2-3 minutes on each side, or until the shrimp are pink and opaque and the vegetables are tender and slightly charred.

7. **Serve:**
   - Remove the skewers from the grill and let them rest for a minute before serving. Enjoy these delicious grilled shrimp and veggie skewers as a light and healthy meal or as part of a larger spread.

Tips:

- For added flavor, you can sprinkle fresh herbs such as parsley or cilantro over the skewers just before serving.
- Serve with a side of quinoa, brown rice, or a fresh green salad to make it a complete meal.
- You can also customize the skewers with your favorite vegetables or even add pineapple chunks for a sweet twist.

5. Turkey and Spinach Stuffed Bell Peppers

Serving Size: 4

Prep Time: 20 minutes

Cooking Time: 30 minutes

Nutrition Information (per serving):

- Calories: 280
- Protein: 25g
- Carbohydrates: 18g
- Dietary Fiber: 6g

- Fat: 12g
- Saturated Fat: 3g
- Sodium: 480mg

Ingredients:

- 4 large bell peppers (any color), tops cut off and seeds removed
- 1 lb ground turkey
- 1 cup fresh spinach, chopped
- 1/2 cup cooked quinoa
- 1/2 cup diced tomatoes (canned or fresh)
- 1/4 cup diced onion
- 2 cloves garlic, minced
- 1/2 cup shredded mozzarella cheese (optional)
- 2 tbsp olive oil
- 1 tsp dried oregano
- 1 tsp dried basil
- Salt and pepper to taste

Directions:

1. **Preheat the Oven:** Preheat your oven to 375°F (190°C).

2. **Prepare the Bell Peppers:** Cut the tops off the bell peppers and remove the seeds and membranes. Set them aside.

3. **Cook the Ground Turkey:** In a large skillet, heat 1 tablespoon of olive oil over medium heat. Add the diced onion and cook until translucent, about 3 minutes. Add the garlic and cook for an additional minute. Add the ground turkey, breaking it up with a spoon, and cook until browned, about 5-7 minutes.

4. **Add Spinach and Seasonings:** Add the chopped spinach to the skillet with the turkey and cook until wilted, about 2 minutes. Stir in the cooked quinoa, diced tomatoes, oregano, basil, salt, and pepper. Cook for another 2-3 minutes until everything is well combined and heated through.

5. **Stuff the Bell Peppers:** Place the bell peppers in a baking dish. Spoon the turkey and spinach mixture into each bell pepper, packing it in tightly.

6. **Bake the Peppers:** Drizzle the remaining olive oil over the stuffed peppers. Cover the baking dish with foil and bake in the preheated oven for 25 minutes. If using, remove the foil, sprinkle the mozzarella cheese on top of the stuffed peppers, and bake for an additional 5 minutes until the cheese is melted and bubbly.

7. **Serve:** Remove the stuffed peppers from the oven and let them cool for a few minutes before serving. Enjoy your healthy and delicious Turkey and Spinach Stuffed Bell Peppers!

Tips for Success:

- **Quinoa Substitute:** If you don't have quinoa, you can substitute it with cooked brown rice or any other whole grain.
- **Vegetarian Option:** For a vegetarian version, replace the ground turkey with a plant-based meat alternative or extra vegetables like mushrooms or zucchini.
- **Extra Flavor:** Add a splash of balsamic vinegar or a squeeze of fresh lemon juice to the turkey mixture for extra flavor.

6. Veggie-Packed Minestrone Soup

Serving Size

This recipe serves 6.

Prep Time

20 minutes

Cooking Time

30 minutes

Nutrition Information (per serving)

- Calories: 180
- Protein: 6g
- Carbohydrates: 28g
- Dietary Fiber: 8g
- Sugars: 7g
- Fat: 5g
- Saturated Fat: 1g
- Sodium: 450mg

Ingredients

- 1 tablespoon olive oil
- 1 large onion, diced
- 2 cloves garlic, minced
- 2 medium carrots, diced
- 2 celery stalks, diced
- 1 zucchini, diced
- 1 yellow squash, diced
- 1 red bell pepper, diced
- 1 can (14.5 oz) diced tomatoes
- 6 cups vegetable broth
- 1 can (15 oz) cannellini beans, drained and rinsed
- 1 cup green beans, trimmed and cut into 1-inch pieces
- 1 cup kale or spinach, chopped
- 1 teaspoon dried oregano
- 1 teaspoon dried basil
- 1/2 teaspoon dried thyme
- Salt and pepper to taste

- 1/2 cup small pasta shells or ditalini (optional)
- Fresh parsley, chopped (for garnish)
- Grated Parmesan cheese (optional, for garnish)

Directions

1. **Heat the Olive Oil**: In a large pot, heat the olive oil over medium heat. Add the diced onion and garlic, and sauté until the onion is translucent, about 5 minutes.
2. **Add the Vegetables**: Stir in the carrots, celery, zucchini, yellow squash, and red bell pepper. Cook for another 5-7 minutes until the vegetables begin to soften.
3. **Add the Tomatoes and Broth**: Pour in the diced tomatoes with their juice and the vegetable broth. Stir to combine.
4. **Add the Beans and Green Beans**: Stir in the cannellini beans and green beans. Add the dried oregano, basil, and thyme. Season with salt and pepper to taste.
5. **Simmer the Soup**: Bring the soup to a boil, then reduce the heat to low. Cover and let it simmer for 15-20 minutes, or until the vegetables are tender.

6. **Add the Greens and Pasta (if using)**: Stir in the chopped kale or spinach. If using pasta, add it to the soup and cook according to the package instructions until al dente, usually about 8-10 minutes.
7. **Adjust Seasoning**: Taste the soup and adjust the seasoning with more salt and pepper if needed.
8. **Serve**: Ladle the soup into bowls. Garnish with fresh parsley and a sprinkle of grated Parmesan cheese, if desired.

CHAPTER 3
DINNER DELIGHTS

1. Grilled Lemon Herb Chicken with Quinoa and Steamed Vegetables

Servings: 4
Prep Time: 20 minutes
Cooking Time: 30 minutes

Nutrition Information (per serving):

- Calories: 350
- Protein: 30g
- Carbohydrates: 35g
- Fat: 10g
- Fiber: 6g

Ingredients:

For the Chicken:

- 4 boneless, skinless chicken breasts
- 2 tbsp olive oil
- 2 tbsp lemon juice
- 2 tsp lemon zest
- 3 cloves garlic, minced

- 1 tsp dried oregano
- 1 tsp dried thyme
- 1 tsp dried rosemary
- Salt and pepper to taste

For the Quinoa:

- 1 cup quinoa
- 2 cups water or low-sodium chicken broth
- 1 tbsp olive oil
- 1 clove garlic, minced
- Salt and pepper to taste

For the Steamed Vegetables:

- 2 cups broccoli florets
- 2 cups carrot slices
- 2 cups green beans, trimmed
- Salt and pepper to taste

Directions:

1. Marinate the Chicken:

- In a small bowl, combine olive oil, lemon juice, lemon zest, minced garlic, oregano, thyme, rosemary, salt, and pepper.
- Place chicken breasts in a resealable plastic bag or shallow dish. Pour the marinade over the chicken, ensuring each piece is well coated.

- Seal the bag or cover the dish and refrigerate for at least 30 minutes, or up to 4 hours for more flavor.

2. Cook the Quinoa:

- Rinse the quinoa under cold water to remove any bitterness.
- In a medium saucepan, heat 1 tablespoon of olive oil over medium heat. Add minced garlic and sauté for about 1 minute until fragrant.
- Add the quinoa and 2 cups of water or chicken broth. Bring to a boil, then reduce the heat to low, cover, and simmer for 15 minutes or until the liquid is absorbed and the quinoa is tender.
- Fluff the quinoa with a fork and season with salt and pepper to taste.

3. Grill the Chicken:

- Preheat your grill to medium-high heat.
- Remove the chicken from the marinade and discard the marinade.
- Grill the chicken for 6-7 minutes per side, or until the internal temperature reaches 165°F (75°C) and the chicken is cooked through.
- Let the chicken rest for a few minutes before slicing.

4. Steam the Vegetables:

- While the chicken is grilling, prepare the steamed vegetables.
- In a large pot with a steamer basket, bring a few inches of water to a boil.
- Add the broccoli, carrots, and green beans to the steamer basket. Cover and steam for about 5-7 minutes until the vegetables are tender but still crisp.
- Season with salt and pepper to taste.

5. Assemble the Dish:

- Divide the cooked quinoa among four plates.
- Arrange a portion of grilled chicken on top of the quinoa.
- Add a generous serving of steamed vegetables on the side.
- Serve immediately and enjoy a healthy, balanced meal!

2. Baked Salmon with Asparagus and Brown Rice

Prep Time: 15 minutes
Cooking Time: 20 minutes
Servings: 4

Ingredients:

- 4 salmon fillets
- 1 bunch asparagus, trimmed
- 2 tbsp olive oil
- 2 cloves garlic, minced
- 1 lemon, sliced
- Salt and pepper to taste
- Fresh dill for garnish (optional)
- 1 cup brown rice
- 2 cups water

Nutrition Information (per serving):

- Calories: 380
- Protein: 34g
- Carbohydrates: 24g
- Fiber: 4g
- Sugars: 2g
- Fat: 16g
- Saturated Fat: 3g
- Cholesterol: 80mg
- Sodium: 150mg

Directions:

1. **Preheat** your oven to 400°F (200°C).
2. **Prepare the Asparagus:**
   - Trim the ends of the asparagus and place them on a baking sheet. Drizzle with 1

tablespoon of olive oil, minced garlic, salt, and pepper. Toss to coat evenly.

3. **Prepare the Salmon:**
   - Place the salmon fillets on the baking sheet with the asparagus. Drizzle the remaining olive oil over the salmon fillets and season with salt and pepper. Place lemon slices on top of each fillet.

4. **Bake:**
   - Bake in the preheated oven for 15-20 minutes, or until the salmon is opaque and flakes easily with a fork.

5. **Cook the Brown Rice:**
   - While the salmon and asparagus are baking, rinse the brown rice under cold water. In a medium saucepan, bring 2 cups of water to a boil. Add the brown rice, reduce heat to low, cover, and simmer for about 15-20 minutes, or until the water is absorbed and the rice is tender.

6. **Serve:**
   - Divide the cooked brown rice among four plates. Top each serving with a baked salmon fillet and a portion of roasted asparagus. Garnish with fresh dill, if desired, and serve hot.

3. Turkey and Zucchini Meatballs with Spaghetti Squash

Prep Time: 20 minutes
Cooking Time: 40 minutes
Servings: 4

Ingredients:

- 1 lb ground turkey
- 1 zucchini, grated and excess moisture squeezed out
- 1/4 cup breadcrumbs (whole wheat or gluten-free)
- 1/4 cup grated Parmesan cheese
- 1 egg
- 2 cloves garlic, minced
- 1 tsp dried oregano
- 1/2 tsp dried basil
- Salt and pepper to taste
- 2 medium spaghetti squashes
- 1 tbsp olive oil
- 1/2 cup marinara sauce (optional)
- Fresh basil leaves, chopped (for garnish)

Nutrition Info (per serving):

- Calories: 320 kcal
- Protein: 30g

- Carbohydrates: 15g
- Fat: 16g
- Fiber: 3g
- Sugar: 4g

Directions:

1. **Prepare Spaghetti Squash:**
   - Preheat oven to 400°F (200°C).
   - Cut spaghetti squashes in half lengthwise and scoop out seeds.
   - Drizzle cut sides with olive oil, salt, and pepper.
   - Place squash halves cut-side down on a baking sheet and roast for 30-40 minutes, until tender. Scrape the flesh with a fork to create spaghetti-like strands.
2. **Make Turkey and Zucchini Meatballs:**
   - In a large bowl, combine ground turkey, grated zucchini, breadcrumbs, Parmesan cheese, egg, garlic, oregano, basil, salt, and pepper. Mix until well combined.
   - Form mixture into meatballs (about 1 inch in diameter).
   - Heat olive oil in a large skillet over medium heat. Add meatballs and cook for 10-12 minutes, turning occasionally, until browned and cooked through.
3. **Serve:**
   - Divide spaghetti squash "rice" among plates.

- o Top with turkey and zucchini meatballs.
- o Optionally, spoon marinara sauce over meatballs.
- o Garnish with chopped fresh basil leaves.
- o Serve hot and enjoy your nutritious and flavorful meal!

4. Stir-Fried Shrimp and Vegetables with Cauliflower Rice

Serving Size: 4
Prep Time: 15 minutes
Cooking Time: 15 minutes
Total Time: 30 minutes

Nutrition Information (per serving):

- Calories: 250 kcal
- Protein: 25g
- Carbohydrates: 15g
- Fiber: 6g
- Sugars: 6g
- Fat: 10g
- Saturated Fat: 1.5g
- Cholesterol: 180mg
- Sodium: 600mg

Ingredients:

- 1 lb large shrimp, peeled and deveined
- 1 head cauliflower, grated into rice-sized pieces
- 1 red bell pepper, thinly sliced
- 1 yellow bell pepper, thinly sliced
- 1 cup snap peas, trimmed
- 1 carrot, julienned
- 3 cloves garlic, minced
- 2 tbsp low-sodium soy sauce
- 1 tbsp sesame oil
- 1 tsp ginger, minced
- 1/4 cup chopped green onions
- Salt and pepper to taste
- Sesame seeds for garnish (optional)

Directions:

1. **Prepare Cauliflower Rice:**
   - Cut the cauliflower into florets and pulse in a food processor until it resembles rice-sized pieces. Alternatively, use pre-riced cauliflower.
2. **Cook Shrimp:**
   - Heat 1 teaspoon of sesame oil in a large skillet or wok over medium-high heat. Add shrimp and cook for 2-3 minutes on each side until pink and opaque. Remove shrimp from skillet and set aside.
3. **Stir-Fry Vegetables:**

- In the same skillet, add remaining sesame oil and garlic. Sauté for 1 minute until fragrant.
- Add bell peppers, snap peas, and carrot. Stir-fry for 3-4 minutes until vegetables are tender-crisp.

4. **Add Cauliflower Rice:**
   - Push vegetables to the side of the skillet and add cauliflower rice. Cook for 2-3 minutes, stirring occasionally, until cauliflower is tender.

5. **Combine Shrimp and Sauce:**
   - Return shrimp to the skillet. Add soy sauce, ginger, and green onions. Stir well to combine and heat through, about 2 minutes.
   - Season with salt and pepper to taste.

6. **Serve:**
   - Divide stir-fried shrimp and vegetables over cauliflower rice among serving plates.
   - Garnish with sesame seeds if desired.
   - Enjoy your flavorful and nutritious Stir-Fried Shrimp and Vegetables with Cauliflower Rice!

5. Quinoa-Stuffed Bell Peppers

Ingredients:

- 4 large bell peppers, tops cut off and seeds removed
- 1 cup cooked quinoa
- 1 cup black beans, drained and rinsed
- 1 cup corn kernels
- 1 cup diced tomatoes
- 1/2 cup shredded low-fat cheese (optional)
- 1 tsp cumin
- 1 tsp paprika
- Salt and pepper to taste
- Fresh cilantro for garnish

Prep Time: 20 minutes
Cooking Time: 30 minutes
Servings: 4

Nutrition Information (per serving):

- Calories: 300
- Protein: 15g
- Carbohydrates: 50g
- Fiber: 10g
- Fat: 5g
- Sodium: 450mg

Directions:

1. **Preheat the Oven:** Preheat your oven to 375°F (190°C).
2. **Prepare the Bell Peppers:** Cut the tops off the bell peppers and remove the seeds. Place them upright in a baking dish.
3. **Prepare the Quinoa Mixture:** In a large mixing bowl, combine the cooked quinoa, black beans, corn kernels, diced tomatoes, cumin, paprika, salt, and pepper. Mix well until all ingredients are evenly distributed.
4. **Stuff the Bell Peppers:** Spoon the quinoa mixture into each bell pepper, packing it tightly and filling them to the top. If desired, sprinkle shredded cheese on top of each stuffed pepper.
5. **Bake:** Cover the baking dish with foil and bake in the preheated oven for 25 minutes. Remove the foil and bake for an additional 5 minutes, or until the bell peppers are tender and the cheese (if using) is melted and bubbly.
6. **Serve:** Garnish with fresh cilantro and serve hot. Each stuffed bell pepper serves as a complete meal, providing a balance of carbohydrates, protein, and fiber to keep you satisfied.

6. Spinach and Mushroom Stuffed Chicken Breast

Serving Size: 4
Prep Time: 20 minutes
Cooking Time: 25 minutes

Ingredients:

- 4 boneless, skinless chicken breasts
- 1 cup baby spinach, chopped
- 1 cup mushrooms, finely chopped
- 1/2 cup shredded mozzarella cheese
- 2 cloves garlic, minced
- 1/2 teaspoon dried thyme
- Salt and pepper to taste
- Olive oil

Directions:

1. **Preheat the oven:** Preheat your oven to 375°F (190°C).
2. **Prepare the filling:** In a skillet, heat a drizzle of olive oil over medium heat. Add minced garlic and sauté for about 1 minute until fragrant. Add chopped mushrooms and cook until softened, about 5-6 minutes. Stir in chopped spinach and cook until wilted. Season with salt, pepper, and

dried thyme. Remove from heat and let cool slightly.

3. **Prepare the chicken breasts:** Lay the chicken breasts flat on a cutting board. Using a sharp knife, cut a pocket into the side of each chicken breast, being careful not to cut all the way through.

4. **Stuff the chicken breasts:** Stuff each chicken breast with the spinach and mushroom mixture, dividing it evenly among the breasts. If needed, secure the openings with toothpicks.

5. **Season the chicken:** Season the stuffed chicken breasts with salt and pepper.

6. **Cook the chicken:** In the same skillet or a new oven-safe skillet, heat a drizzle of olive oil over medium-high heat. Add the stuffed chicken breasts and sear for about 3-4 minutes on each side until golden brown.

7. **Bake:** Transfer the skillet to the preheated oven and bake for 15-20 minutes, or until the chicken reaches an internal temperature of 165°F (74°C) and is cooked through.

8. **Serve:** Remove the toothpicks (if used) before serving. Optionally, sprinkle with shredded mozzarella cheese over each chicken breast during the last 5 minutes of baking for a cheesy topping.

Nutrition Information (per serving):

- **Calories:** 280 kcal
- **Protein:** 40g
- **Carbohydrates:** 4g

- **Fat:** 11g
- **Saturated Fat:** 4g
- **Cholesterol:** 120mg
- **Sodium:** 300mg
- **Fiber:** 1g
- **Sugar:** 1g

CHAPTER 4

SNACKS AND APPETIZERS

1. Greek Yogurt and Berry Parfait

Prep Time: 10 minutes
Servings: 2

Nutrition per Serving:

- Calories: 180 kcal
- Protein: 12g
- Carbohydrates: 30g
- Fat: 2g
- Fiber: 5g

Ingredients:

- 1 cup Greek yogurt (plain or vanilla)
- 1 cup mixed berries (such as strawberries, blueberries, raspberries)
- 1/4 cup granola
- 1 tbsp honey (optional, for drizzling)
- Fresh mint leaves for garnish (optional)

Directions:

1. **Prepare the Berries:**
   - Rinse the berries under cold water and pat dry with a paper towel.
   - If using strawberries, hull them and slice into halves or quarters.
2. **Assemble the Parfait:**
   - In two serving glasses or bowls, start by layering a spoonful of Greek yogurt at the bottom.
3. **Add Berries and Granola:**
   - Top the yogurt with a layer of mixed berries, distributing them evenly.
   - Sprinkle a layer of granola over the berries. You can use homemade or store-bought granola for added crunch and flavor.
4. **Repeat Layers:**
   - Repeat the layers of Greek yogurt, berries, and granola until the glasses are filled or you run out of ingredients. Ensure the top layer is yogurt.
5. **Drizzle with Honey (Optional):**
   - For added sweetness, drizzle honey over the top layer of yogurt.
6. **Garnish and Serve:**
   - Garnish with fresh mint leaves for a pop of color and freshness.
   - Serve immediately and enjoy your nutritious Greek Yogurt and Berry Parfait!

Tips:

- Customize your parfait by using different types of berries or adding sliced bananas or peaches.
- For a dairy-free version, substitute Greek yogurt with coconut yogurt or almond milk yogurt.
- Prepare the parfaits ahead of time and refrigerate them for up to 2 hours before serving to allow the flavors to meld together.

2. Avocado and Hummus Stuffed Mini Peppers

Serving Size: Makes 12 stuffed mini peppers
Prep Time: 15 minutes
Cooking Time: 0 minutes
Total Time: 15 minutes

Nutrition Information (per serving):

- **Calories:** 65 kcal
- **Total Fat:** 4.5 g
- **Saturated Fat:** 0.7 g
- **Cholesterol:** 0 mg
- **Sodium:** 65 mg
- **Total Carbohydrates:** 6.3 g
- **Dietary Fiber:** 2.3 g

- **Total Sugars:** 2.1 g
- **Protein:** 1.8 g

Ingredients:

- 12 mini sweet peppers, halved and deseeded
- 1 ripe avocado
- Juice of 1/2 lemon
- 1/2 cup hummus (store-bought or homemade)
- Salt and pepper to taste
- Fresh parsley or cilantro for garnish (optional)

Directions:

1. **Prepare the Mini Peppers:**
   - Wash the mini peppers thoroughly. Slice them in half lengthwise and remove the seeds and membranes using a small spoon or knife. Set aside.
2. **Make the Avocado Filling:**
   - Cut the avocado in half, remove the pit, and scoop the flesh into a bowl. Mash the avocado with a fork until smooth. Add lemon juice, salt, and pepper to taste, and mix well.
3. **Stuff the Peppers:**
   - Spoon hummus into each mini pepper half, filling them about halfway.
   - Top each pepper with a dollop of mashed avocado mixture, spreading it evenly over the hummus.

4. **Garnish and Serve:**
   - Garnish with fresh parsley or cilantro if desired.
   - Arrange stuffed mini peppers on a serving platter and serve immediately.

Tips:

- Choose mini peppers that are firm and brightly colored for the best flavor and presentation.
- Customize the hummus by using different flavors such as roasted red pepper or garlic for added variety.
- These stuffed mini peppers can be prepared ahead of time and stored in the refrigerator for up to 2 days. Garnish just before serving to maintain freshness.

3. Cucumber and Smoked Salmon Bites

Serving Size: Makes 12 bites
Prep Time: 15 minutes
Cooking Time: 0 minutes

Ingredients:

- 1 English cucumber
- 4 oz smoked salmon, thinly sliced
- 1/4 cup cream cheese or Greek yogurt
- 1 tbsp fresh dill, chopped
- 1 tbsp capers (optional)
- Salt and pepper to taste

Directions:

1. **Prepare the Cucumber:**
   - Wash the cucumber and cut it into 1/2-inch thick slices. You should get about 12 slices from one cucumber. If desired, you can peel stripes of skin off the cucumber for a decorative effect.
2. **Prepare the Topping:**
   - In a small bowl, mix together the cream cheese (or Greek yogurt) with chopped fresh dill. Season with salt and pepper to taste.
3. **Assemble the Bites:**
   - Place a small dollop of the cream cheese mixture on top of each cucumber slice.
4. **Add Smoked Salmon:**
   - Carefully fold or twist a slice of smoked salmon and place it on top of the cream cheese.
5. **Garnish:**
   - If using, top each bite with a caper and a sprig of fresh dill.
6. **Serve:**

- o Arrange the cucumber and smoked salmon bites on a serving platter and serve immediately. These bites can be enjoyed as an elegant appetizer or a light snack.

Nutrition Information (per bite):

- Calories: 30 kcal
- Protein: 3g
- Fat: 1.5g
- Carbohydrates: 1g
- Fiber: 0.5g
- Sugar: 0.5g
- Sodium: 120mg

Tips:

- Ensure the cucumber slices are thick enough to hold the toppings without breaking.
- Adjust the amount of cream cheese or Greek yogurt to your preference for creaminess.
- For added flavor, you can sprinkle a pinch of lemon zest over the bites before serving.

4. Baked Zucchini Fries

Serving Size: 4 servings
Prep Time: 15 minutes

Cooking Time: 20 minutes
Total Time: 35 minutes

Ingredients:

- 2 medium zucchinis
- 1/2 cup panko breadcrumbs
- 1/4 cup grated Parmesan cheese
- 1/2 tsp garlic powder
- 1/2 tsp paprika
- 1/4 tsp salt
- 1/4 tsp black pepper
- 1/4 cup all-purpose flour
- 2 large eggs, beaten
- Cooking spray or olive oil spray

Nutrition Information (per serving):

- Calories: 120 kcal
- Protein: 7g
- Carbohydrates: 15g
- Fat: 4g
- Saturated Fat: 1.5g
- Fiber: 2g
- Sugar: 3g
- Sodium: 310mg

Directions:

1. **Preheat the Oven:** Preheat your oven to 425°F (220°C). Line a baking sheet with parchment paper and lightly coat it with cooking spray.
2. **Prepare the Zucchini:** Wash the zucchinis thoroughly and cut them into thin strips, resembling the shape of fries.
3. **Set Up Your Dredging Station:**
   o In a shallow bowl or dish, place the all-purpose flour.
   o In another shallow bowl, beat the eggs until well combined.
   o In a third shallow bowl, mix together the panko breadcrumbs, Parmesan cheese, garlic powder, paprika, salt, and black pepper.
4. **Dredge the Zucchini Strips:**
   o Coat each zucchini strip in the flour, shaking off any excess.
   o Dip it into the beaten egg, allowing any excess to drip off.
   o Press the zucchini strip into the breadcrumb mixture, ensuring it is evenly coated.
5. **Arrange on Baking Sheet:** Place each coated zucchini strip onto the prepared baking sheet in a single layer. Leave a little space between each strip to ensure they bake evenly.
6. **Bake:** Lightly spray the tops of the zucchini fries with cooking spray or olive oil spray to help them crisp up in the oven. Bake for 18-20 minutes,

flipping halfway through, until the fries are golden brown and crispy.

7. **Serve:** Remove from the oven and let them cool slightly before serving. Enjoy your baked zucchini fries with your favorite dipping sauce, such as marinara sauce, ranch dressing, or a yogurt-based dip.

Tips:

- For extra crispiness, you can place a wire rack on top of the baking sheet and arrange the zucchini fries on the rack.
- Experiment with different seasonings such as Italian seasoning, cayenne pepper, or lemon zest to customize the flavor to your liking.
- These fries are best enjoyed immediately after baking for optimal crispiness.

5. Spicy Roasted Chickpeas

Prep Time: 5 minutes
Cooking Time: 30 minutes
Servings: 4

Ingredients:

- 2 cans (15 oz each) chickpeas (garbanzo beans), drained, rinsed, and patted dry
- 2 tbsp olive oil
- 1 tsp smoked paprika
- 1/2 tsp cayenne pepper (adjust to taste for spiciness)
- 1/2 tsp garlic powder
- 1/2 tsp salt
- Freshly ground black pepper to taste

Nutrition Information (per serving):

- Calories: 180 kcal
- Total Fat: 7g
- Saturated Fat: 1g
- Sodium: 380mg
- Total Carbohydrates: 23g
- Dietary Fiber: 6g
- Sugars: 1g
- Protein: 7g

Directions:

1. **Preheat Oven and Prep Chickpeas**
   - Preheat your oven to 400°F (200°C). Line a baking sheet with parchment paper for easy cleanup.

o Drain and rinse the chickpeas thoroughly. Pat them dry with a kitchen towel to remove excess moisture.

2. **Season Chickpeas**
   o In a large bowl, toss the chickpeas with olive oil, smoked paprika, cayenne pepper, garlic powder, salt, and black pepper until evenly coated. Adjust the amount of cayenne pepper to suit your spice preference.

3. **Roast Chickpeas**
   o Spread the seasoned chickpeas in a single layer on the prepared baking sheet.
   o Roast in the preheated oven for 25-30 minutes, shaking the pan halfway through cooking, until the chickpeas are golden brown and crispy.

4. **Cool and Serve**
   o Remove from the oven and let the chickpeas cool slightly on the baking sheet before transferring them to a serving bowl.
   o Enjoy warm or at room temperature as a crunchy snack or salad topper.

Tips:

- Ensure the chickpeas are thoroughly dried after rinsing to achieve maximum crispiness.
- Experiment with different seasonings like curry powder, cumin, or chili powder for varied flavors.

- Store any leftovers in an airtight container at room temperature for up to 3 days, though they are best enjoyed fresh.

6. Caprese Skewers

Serving Size: Makes about 12 skewers
Prep Time: 15 minutes
Cooking Time: 0 minutes

Ingredients:

- 12 cherry or grape tomatoes
- 12 small fresh mozzarella balls (bocconcini)
- 12 fresh basil leaves
- Balsamic glaze, for drizzling (optional)
- Salt and pepper, to taste
- Wooden skewers or toothpicks

Directions:

1. **Prepare the Ingredients:**
   o Rinse the cherry or grape tomatoes and pat them dry.
   o Drain the fresh mozzarella balls if they are stored in liquid.
   o Wash and dry the fresh basil leaves.
2. **Assemble the Skewers:**

- Take a wooden skewer or toothpick and thread on one cherry tomato, followed by a fresh basil leaf folded in half, and then a mozzarella ball.
- Repeat with the remaining ingredients until you have assembled all 12 skewers.

3. **Season and Garnish:**
   - Once assembled, lightly season the skewers with salt and pepper to taste.
   - Optionally, drizzle balsamic glaze over the skewers for added flavor and presentation.

4. **Serve:**
   - Arrange the Caprese skewers on a serving platter or board.
   - They can be served immediately as a cold appetizer or at room temperature.

Nutrition Information (per serving):

- Calories: 60 kcal
- Total Fat: 3.5 g
  - Saturated Fat: 2 g
- Cholesterol: 10 mg
- Sodium: 120 mg
- Total Carbohydrates: 2 g
  - Dietary Fiber: 0 g
  - Sugars: 1 g
- Protein: 5 g

CHAPTER 5

DESSERTS AND SWEET TREATS

1. Greek Yogurt Parfait with Berries and Honey

Serving Size: 1 parfait
Prep Time: 5 minutes
Cooking Time: 0 minutes

Ingredients:

- 1/2 cup Greek yogurt
- 1/2 cup mixed berries (such as strawberries, blueberries, raspberries)
- 1 tbsp honey
- 2 tbsp granola (optional, for topping)

Nutrition Information (per serving):

- Calories: 200 kcal
- Protein: 14g
- Carbohydrates: 30g
- Fat: 4g
- Fiber: 4g
- Sugar: 24g
- Sodium: 60mg

Directions:

1. **Prepare the Yogurt:** Spoon Greek yogurt into a serving bowl or glass.
2. **Add Berries:** Wash and dry the berries. Slice any larger berries like strawberries.
3. **Layer the Parfait:** Begin by adding a layer of Greek yogurt to the bottom of the bowl or glass. Top with a layer of mixed berries.
4. **Drizzle with Honey:** Drizzle honey evenly over the berries.
5. **Repeat Layers:** Repeat the layers of Greek yogurt, berries, and honey until the bowl or glass is full.
6. **Optional Topping:** Sprinkle granola on top for added crunch and texture.
7. **Serve Immediately:** Enjoy your Greek Yogurt Parfait fresh or refrigerate until ready to serve.

Tips:

- Customize your parfait by adding different fruits or nuts.

- For a vegan option, use dairy-free yogurt and substitute maple syrup for honey.

2. Chia Seed Pudding

Serving Size: 2
Prep Time: 5 minutes
Cooking Time: 0 minutes

Ingredients:

- 1/4 cup chia seeds
- 1 cup unsweetened almond milk (or any milk of choice)
- 1 tbsp maple syrup or honey (optional, for sweetness)
- 1/2 tsp vanilla extract
- Fresh fruits or nuts for topping (optional)

Nutrition Info (per serving):

- Calories: 150
- Total Fat: 8g
- Saturated Fat: 1g
- Cholesterol: 0mg
- Sodium: 80mg
- Total Carbohydrates: 15g
- Dietary Fiber: 10g
- Sugars: 4g
- Protein: 6g

Directions:

1. **Mix Ingredients:** In a bowl or jar, combine chia seeds, almond milk, maple syrup (if using), and vanilla extract. Stir well until all ingredients are fully combined.
2. **Set Aside:** Let the mixture sit for 5 minutes, then stir again to break up any clumps of chia seeds. Cover the bowl or jar and refrigerate for at least 2 hours, or preferably overnight.
3. **Serve:** Once the chia seeds have absorbed the liquid and formed a pudding-like consistency, give it a final stir. If desired, top with fresh fruits or nuts before serving.
4. **Enjoy:** Spoon into serving bowls or jars and enjoy this nutritious and satisfying chia seed pudding!

Tips:

- For a creamier texture, blend the mixture after refrigerating for a smoother pudding.
- Experiment with different toppings such as berries, sliced bananas, shredded coconut, or cocoa nibs.
- Adjust sweetness by adding more or less maple syrup or honey according to your taste preferences.

3. Baked Apple Slices with Cinnamon

Prep Time: 10 minutes
Cooking Time: 20 minutes
Servings: 4

Ingredients:

- 4 medium apples (such as Granny Smith or Honeycrisp), cored and thinly sliced
- 2 tbsp melted butter or coconut oil
- 1 tbsp honey or maple syrup (optional, for added sweetness)
- 1 tsp ground cinnamon
- Pinch of nutmeg (optional)
- Pinch of salt

Nutrition Information (per serving):

- Calories: 120
- Total Fat: 4g
- Saturated Fat: 3g
- Cholesterol: 10mg
- Sodium: 35mg
- Total Carbohydrate: 23g
- Dietary Fiber: 4g
- Sugars: 17g
- Protein: 0.5g

Directions:

1. **Preheat** your oven to 375°F (190°C). Line a baking sheet with parchment paper or lightly grease it.
2. **Prepare** the apples by coring and thinly slicing them. Place the apple slices in a large bowl.
3. **Mix** together the melted butter or coconut oil, honey or maple syrup (if using), cinnamon, nutmeg (if using), and a pinch of salt in a small bowl.
4. **Coat** the apple slices evenly with the cinnamon mixture. Toss gently to ensure all slices are coated.
5. **Arrange** the coated apple slices in a single layer on the prepared baking sheet.
6. **Bake** in the preheated oven for 15-20 minutes, or until the apples are tender and lightly caramelized, stirring halfway through cooking.
7. **Serve** warm as a delicious and healthy dessert or snack option. Optionally, garnish with a sprinkle of additional cinnamon before serving.

4. Dark Chocolate Avocado Mousse

Prep Time: 10 minutes
Cooking Time: 0 minutes
Servings: 4

Nutrition Information (per serving):

- Calories: 210 kcal
- Protein: 3g
- Fat: 16g
- Carbohydrates: 17g
- Fiber: 7g
- Sugar: 6g
- Sodium: 5mg

Ingredients:

- 2 ripe avocados, peeled and pitted
- 1/4 cup unsweetened cocoa powder
- 1/4 cup maple syrup or honey (adjust to taste)
- 1 tsp vanilla extract
- Pinch of salt
- Optional toppings: fresh berries, shaved dark chocolate, whipped cream

Directions:

1. **Prepare the Avocado:**
   - In a food processor or blender, add the peeled and pitted avocados.
2. **Blend Ingredients:**
   - Add cocoa powder, maple syrup or honey, vanilla extract, and a pinch of salt to the avocados.

3. **Blend Until Smooth:**
   - Blend until the mixture is smooth and creamy, scraping down the sides as needed to ensure all ingredients are well combined.
4. **Chill (Optional):**
   - For a thicker consistency, chill the mousse in the refrigerator for 30 minutes before serving.
5. **Serve:**
   - Divide the mousse into serving dishes.
   - Garnish with fresh berries, shaved dark chocolate, or a dollop of whipped cream if desired.
6. **Enjoy:**
   - Serve immediately and enjoy the rich, chocolatey flavor of this decadent yet healthy dessert!

5. Banana Oat Cookies

Servings: Makes about 12 cookies
Prep Time: 10 minutes
Cooking Time: 15 minutes
Total Time: 25 minutes

Nutrition per Serving:

Calories: 120 kcal, Fat: 4g, Carbohydrates: 20g, Fiber: 2g, Protein: 2g

Ingredients:

- 2 ripe bananas, mashed
- 1 cup rolled oats
- 1/4 cup almond butter or peanut butter
- 1/4 cup raisins or chocolate chips (optional)
- 1/2 tsp vanilla extract
- 1/2 tsp cinnamon
- Pinch of salt

Directions:

1. **Preheat** your oven to 350°F (175°C). Line a baking sheet with parchment paper or lightly grease it.
2. **Mix Ingredients:** In a large bowl, combine the mashed bananas, rolled oats, almond or peanut butter, optional raisins or chocolate chips, vanilla extract, cinnamon, and a pinch of salt. Stir until all ingredients are well combined.
3. **Form Cookies:** Drop spoonfuls of the cookie dough onto the prepared baking sheet, spacing them about 2 inches apart. Use the back of the spoon or your fingers to gently flatten each cookie.
4. **Bake:** Place the baking sheet in the preheated oven and bake for 15 minutes, or until the cookies are lightly golden brown on the edges.

5. **Cool and Enjoy:** Remove the cookies from the oven and let them cool on the baking sheet for 5 minutes. Transfer to a wire rack to cool completely before serving. Enjoy these healthy and delicious banana oat cookies as a nutritious snack or quick breakfast option!

6. Coconut Milk Rice Pudding

Serving Size: 4
Prep Time: 5 minutes
Cooking Time: 30 minutes

Ingredients:

- 1 cup jasmine rice
- 2 cups coconut milk
- 1/2 cup water
- 1/4 cup sugar (adjust to taste)
- 1/4 tsp salt
- 1 tsp vanilla extract
- Optional toppings: Fresh berries, toasted coconut flakes, or nuts for garnish

Directions:

1. **Rinse the Rice:** Rinse the jasmine rice under cold water until the water runs clear. This helps remove excess starch for a creamier pudding.

2. **Combine Ingredients:** In a medium saucepan, combine the rinsed rice, coconut milk, water, sugar, salt, and vanilla extract. Stir well to dissolve the sugar and salt.
3. **Cook the Rice:** Bring the mixture to a gentle boil over medium-high heat, stirring occasionally to prevent the rice from sticking to the bottom of the pan.
4. **Simmer:** Once boiling, reduce the heat to low and cover the saucepan with a lid. Let the rice simmer for 20-25 minutes, or until the rice is tender and the liquid has been absorbed. Stir occasionally to ensure even cooking.
5. **Serve:** Remove the saucepan from heat and let the rice pudding cool slightly before serving. Serve warm or chilled, garnished with fresh berries, toasted coconut flakes, or nuts if desired.

Nutrition Information (per serving):

- Calories: 320 kcal
- Total Fat: 18g
  - Saturated Fat: 16g
  - Trans Fat: 0g
- Cholesterol: 0mg
- Sodium: 150mg
- Total Carbohydrates: 36g
  - Dietary Fiber: 2g
  - Sugars: 12g
- Protein: 4g

Notes:

- **Storage:** Store any leftovers in an airtight container in the refrigerator for up to 3 days. Reheat gently before serving.
- **Variations:** Experiment with different toppings such as mango slices, cinnamon, or a drizzle of honey for added flavor.

CHAPTER 6

DRINKS AND SMOOTHIES

1. Green Detox Smoothie

Serving Size: 1
Prep Time: 5 minutes
Cooking Time: None

Nutrition Information (per serving):

- **Calories:** 180 kcal
- **Carbohydrates:** 35 g
- **Protein:** 5 g
- **Fat:** 3 g
- **Fiber:** 8 g
- **Sugar:** 20 g
- **Vitamin A:** 150% DV
- **Vitamin C:** 80% DV
- **Calcium:** 15% DV
- **Iron:** 10% DV

Ingredients:

- 1 cup spinach, packed
- 1/2 cup cucumber, chopped
- 1/2 avocado, pitted and peeled
- 1 small apple, cored and chopped
- 1/2 lemon, juiced
- 1 tbsp fresh ginger, grated
- 1 cup unsweetened almond milk (or any preferred milk)
- 1 tbsp chia seeds
- Ice cubes (optional)

Directions:

1. **Prepare Ingredients:**
   - Wash the spinach thoroughly.
   - Peel and chop the cucumber.
   - Pit and peel the avocado.
   - Core and chop the apple.
   - Juice the lemon.
   - Grate the fresh ginger.
2. **Blend Ingredients:**
   - In a blender, combine spinach, cucumber, avocado, apple, lemon juice, ginger, almond milk, and chia seeds.
   - Add a handful of ice cubes if desired for a colder smoothie.
3. **Blend Until Smooth:**
   - Blend on high until the mixture is smooth and creamy, about 1-2 minutes. Scrape

down the sides of the blender if needed and blend again.

4. **Serve:**
   - Pour the Green Detox Smoothie into a glass.
   - Garnish with a slice of cucumber or a sprig of mint, if desired.
   - Enjoy immediately to benefit from its freshness and nutritional value.

Tip: You can customize this smoothie by adding a scoop of protein powder for an extra boost of protein, or swap out ingredients based on your taste preferences and dietary needs.

2. Berry Protein Smoothie

Serving Size: 1 smoothie
Prep Time: 5 minutes
Cooking Time: 0 minutes

Ingredients:

- 1/2 cup mixed berries (strawberries, blueberries, raspberries)
- 1/2 banana, sliced
- 1/2 cup plain Greek yogurt
- 1/2 cup almond milk (or any milk of your choice)

- 1 scoop vanilla protein powder
- 1 tbsp honey (optional, for added sweetness)
- Ice cubes (optional, for desired consistency)

Nutrition Information:

- Calories: 250
- Protein: 25g
- Carbohydrates: 30g
- Fat: 3g
- Fiber: 5g
- Sugar: 20g
- Vitamin C: 60% DV
- Calcium: 20% DV
- Iron: 8% DV

Directions:

1. **Prepare Ingredients:** Gather all the ingredients needed for the smoothie.
2. **Blend Ingredients:** In a blender, combine the mixed berries, sliced banana, Greek yogurt, almond milk, vanilla protein powder, and honey (if using).
3. **Blend Until Smooth:** Blend on high until the mixture is smooth and creamy. If desired, add ice cubes to achieve the desired consistency and blend again briefly.
4. **Serve:** Pour the smoothie into a glass and enjoy immediately for a refreshing and nutritious boost!

Tips:

- For a thicker smoothie, use frozen berries or add more ice cubes.
- Adjust sweetness by adding more or less honey, depending on your taste preferences.
- Customize your smoothie by adding spinach or kale for extra nutrients without altering the berry flavor.

3. Refreshing Cucumber Mint Water

Serving Size: 1 pitcher
Prep Time: 5 minutes
Cooking Time: 0 minutes

Nutrition Info: (Per serving)

- Calories: 0
- Carbohydrates: 0g
- Fiber: 0g
- Sugar: 0g
- Protein: 0g
- Fat: 0g
- Sodium: 0mg

Ingredients:

- 1 medium cucumber, thinly sliced
- 10-12 fresh mint leaves
- Ice cubes
- Water (enough to fill the pitcher)

Directions:

1. **Prepare the Ingredients:**
   - Wash the cucumber thoroughly and slice it thinly. Rinse the mint leaves under cold water.
2. **Assemble the Drink:**
   - In a large pitcher, combine the sliced cucumber and fresh mint leaves.
3. **Add Water:**
   - Fill the pitcher with cold water, leaving some space at the top for ice cubes.
4. **Chill:**
   - Place the pitcher in the refrigerator for at least 1 hour to allow the flavors to infuse.
5. **Serve:**
   - When ready to serve, add ice cubes to the pitcher to chill the water further.
6. **Enjoy:**
   - Pour the cucumber mint water into glasses filled with ice cubes. Garnish with additional cucumber slices or mint leaves if desired. Serve and enjoy this refreshing and hydrating drink!

Tips:

- For a stronger flavor, muddle the mint leaves slightly before adding them to the pitcher.
- You can adjust the intensity of the flavors by letting the water infuse for a longer period.
- This drink is perfect for staying hydrated on hot days and can be a delightful addition to any meal or as a standalone refreshment.

4. Turmeric Ginger Tea

Serving Size: 1 cup
Prep Time: 5 minutes
Cooking Time: 10 minutes

Ingredients:

- 1 cup water
- 1/2 teaspoon ground turmeric (or 1-inch fresh turmeric root, grated)
- 1/2 teaspoon ground ginger (or 1-inch fresh ginger root, grated)
- 1 teaspoon honey (optional)
- Juice of 1/2 lemon (optional)
- Pinch of black pepper (enhances turmeric absorption)
- Fresh mint leaves for garnish (optional)

Nutrition Information (per serving):

- Calories: 10 kcal

- Carbohydrates: 2 g
- Fiber: 0.5 g
- Protein: 0.2 g
- Fat: 0.1 g
- Sodium: 1 mg

Directions:

1. **Prepare the Ingredients:**
   - If using fresh turmeric and ginger, peel and grate them. Set aside.
   - Juice half a lemon and set aside.
2. **Boil the Water:**
   - In a small saucepan, bring 1 cup of water to a boil.
3. **Brew the Tea:**
   - Add the grated turmeric and ginger (or ground turmeric and ginger) to the boiling water.
   - Reduce heat to low and let it simmer for 8-10 minutes to extract flavors.
4. **Strain and Serve:**
   - Remove from heat and strain the tea into a cup using a fine mesh strainer.
   - Add honey and lemon juice to taste, if desired.
   - Sprinkle with a pinch of black pepper.
5. **Garnish and Enjoy:**
   - Garnish with fresh mint leaves for added freshness and aroma, if desired.

- o Serve hot and enjoy the soothing and nutritious benefits of turmeric ginger tea!

Benefits of Turmeric Ginger Tea:

- **Anti-inflammatory:** Both turmeric and ginger are known for their anti-inflammatory properties, which may help reduce inflammation in the body.
- **Digestive Aid:** Ginger can aid digestion and alleviate nausea.
- **Immune Support:** Turmeric and ginger have antioxidants that support the immune system.

5. Matcha Green Tea Latte

Serving Size: 1 latte
Prep Time: 5 minutes
Cooking Time: 5 minutes
Total Time: 10 minutes

Nutrition Information (per serving):

- **Calories:** 80 kcal
- **Protein:** 3g
- **Fat:** 3g
- **Carbohydrates:** 12g
- **Fiber:** 1g
- **Sugar:** 8g

- **Sodium:** 80mg

Ingredients:

- 1 tsp matcha green tea powder
- 1 tbsp hot water (not boiling)
- 1 cup unsweetened almond milk (or milk of your choice)
- 1 tsp honey or sweetener of choice (optional)
- Ice cubes (optional)

Directions:

1. **Prepare the Matcha:** In a small bowl or cup, sift the matcha green tea powder to remove any clumps. Add 1 tablespoon of hot water (around 175°F or 80°C). Whisk vigorously with a bamboo whisk or a small whisk until the matcha is fully dissolved and frothy.
2. **Heat the Milk:** In a small saucepan, heat the almond milk (or milk of your choice) over medium heat until steaming hot. Do not boil.
3. **Combine and Sweeten:** Pour the steamed milk into a mug. Add the dissolved matcha green tea to the milk. Stir in honey or sweetener to taste, if desired.
4. **Optional Iced Latte:** For an iced latte, allow the matcha mixture to cool after step 3. Fill a glass with ice cubes and pour the matcha mixture over the ice.

5. **Serve:** Stir gently to combine and enjoy your homemade matcha green tea latte!

Tips:

- Adjust the sweetness by adding more or less honey or sweetener.
- For a creamier latte, use frothed milk or add a splash of coconut cream.
- Experiment with different milk alternatives such as oat milk or soy milk for variety.

Benefits of Matcha Green Tea Latte:

- Matcha is rich in antioxidants and provides a gentle caffeine boost.
- It may help boost metabolism and promote calmness due to its L-theanine content.
- Enjoy as a healthier alternative to traditional coffee-based lattes.

6. Spiced Apple Cider

Prep Time: 5 minutes
Cooking Time: 20 minutes
Servings: 4

Ingredients:

- 4 cups apple cider
- 1/2 cup water
- 2 cinnamon sticks
- 4 whole cloves
- 1/2 teaspoon whole allspice berries
- 1/4 teaspoon ground nutmeg
- 1/4 cup brown sugar (optional, adjust sweetness to taste)
- Orange slices or cinnamon sticks for garnish (optional)

Directions:

1. **Combine Ingredients:** In a medium-sized pot, combine apple cider, water, cinnamon sticks, cloves, allspice berries, and ground nutmeg. Add brown sugar if desired for added sweetness.
2. **Simmer:** Bring the mixture to a simmer over medium heat. Reduce heat to low and let it simmer gently for 15-20 minutes to allow the spices to infuse into the cider. Stir occasionally.
3. **Strain and Serve:** After simmering, remove the pot from heat. Using a fine mesh sieve or cheesecloth, strain out the spices and discard them.
4. **Serve:** Ladle the spiced apple cider into mugs or heatproof glasses. Garnish each serving with an orange slice or cinnamon stick if desired. Serve hot and enjoy!

Nutrition Information (per serving):

- Calories: 120 kcal
- Carbohydrates: 30 g
- Fat: 0 g
- Protein: 0 g
- Fiber: 0 g
- Sugar: 25 g
- Sodium: 10 mg

Tips:

- For a stronger spice flavor, allow the cider to simmer for a longer period.
- Adjust sweetness by adding more or less brown sugar according to your preference.
- Serve with a cinnamon stick in each mug for an extra touch of flavor.

CHAPTER 7

MEAL PLANNING AND PREP

1. Grilled Chicken and Quinoa Salad

Servings: 6
Prep Time: 10 minutes
Cooking Time: 30 minutes

Nutrition Information (per serving):

- **Calories:** 120
- **Total Fat:** 0g
- **Sodium:** 5mg
- **Total Carbohydrates:** 30g
- **Sugars:** 26g
- **Protein:** 0g

Ingredients:

- 8 cups apple cider
- 1 orange, thinly sliced
- 4 cinnamon sticks
- 6 whole cloves
- 4 whole allspice berries

- 1-inch piece fresh ginger, sliced
- 1/4 teaspoon ground nutmeg
- 2 tablespoons brown sugar (optional)
- 1/4 cup fresh cranberries (optional, for garnish)
- 2 tablespoons honey (optional, for added sweetness)

Directions:

1. **Prepare the Spices:** In a large pot, combine the apple cider, orange slices, cinnamon sticks, cloves, allspice berries, sliced ginger, and ground nutmeg.
2. **Simmer the Cider:** Place the pot over medium heat and bring the mixture to a simmer. Reduce the heat to low and let it simmer for about 30 minutes, allowing the flavors to meld together.
3. **Taste and Adjust:** After 30 minutes, taste the cider. If you prefer a sweeter drink, add the brown sugar and honey, stirring until dissolved. Adjust the sweetness to your liking.
4. **Strain and Serve:** Strain the cider to remove the spices and orange slices. Pour the spiced cider into mugs, garnish with fresh cranberries if desired, and serve warm.

Tips:

- For an extra kick, add a splash of rum or bourbon to each mug before serving.

- Leftover spiced cider can be stored in the refrigerator for up to a week and reheated as needed.

2. Baked Salmon with Asparagus

Servings: 4
Prep Time: 15 minutes
Cooking Time: 20 minutes

Nutrition Information (per serving):

- Calories: 350
- Protein: 30g
- Fat: 20g
- Carbohydrates: 10g
- Fiber: 4g

Ingredients:

- 4 salmon fillets
- 1 bunch asparagus, trimmed
- 2 tbsp olive oil
- 2 cloves garlic, minced
- 1 lemon, sliced
- Salt and pepper to taste
- Fresh dill for garnish (optional)

Directions:

1. **Preheat the Oven:** Preheat your oven to 400°F (200°C) to ensure it's hot and ready when you need to bake the salmon and asparagus.
2. **Prepare the Asparagus:** Toss the asparagus spears with 1 tablespoon of olive oil, minced garlic, salt, and pepper. Arrange them in a single layer on a baking sheet.
3. **Season the Salmon:** Place the salmon fillets on the baking sheet next to the asparagus. Drizzle the fillets with the remaining olive oil and season with salt and pepper. Top each fillet with a lemon slice to add a refreshing citrus flavor.
4. **Bake:** Place the baking sheet in the preheated oven and bake for 15-20 minutes. The salmon is done when it is opaque and flakes easily with a fork, and the asparagus should be tender but still crisp.
5. **Serve:** Remove from the oven and let the salmon rest for a few minutes. Garnish with fresh dill if desired, and serve immediately.

Tips for Success:

- **Choose Fresh Salmon:** Opt for fresh, wild-caught salmon if possible, as it has a richer flavor and higher nutritional value.

- **Don't Overcook:** Keep an eye on the salmon as it bakes. Overcooked salmon can become dry and lose its delicate texture.
- **Add Variety:** For an extra burst of flavor, try adding a sprinkle of your favorite herbs or a dash of balsamic vinegar before baking.

3. Turkey and Vegetable Stir-Fry

Serving Size

- **Servings:** 4

Cooking Time

- **Prep Time:** 15 minutes
- **Cooking Time:** 15 minutes

Nutrition Information (per serving)

- **Calories:** 280
- **Protein:** 26g
- **Carbohydrates:** 14g
- **Dietary Fiber:** 4g
- **Sugars:** 7g
- **Fat:** 12g
- **Saturated Fat:** 2g

- **Cholesterol:** 85mg
- **Sodium:** 550mg

Ingredients

- 1 lb ground turkey
- 1 red bell pepper, sliced
- 1 yellow bell pepper, sliced
- 1 zucchini, sliced
- 1 carrot, julienned
- 1 cup snap peas
- 2 tbsp soy sauce (low sodium)
- 1 tbsp hoisin sauce
- 1 tbsp olive oil
- 2 cloves garlic, minced
- 1 tsp ginger, minced

Directions

1. **Cook the Turkey:**
   - In a large skillet, heat olive oil over medium heat. Add ground turkey and cook until browned, breaking it apart with a spoon.
2. **Add Vegetables:**
   - Add garlic and ginger to the skillet and cook for 1 minute. Then add bell peppers, zucchini, carrot, and snap

peas. Stir-fry for 5-7 minutes, until vegetables are tender-crisp.

3. **Add Sauces:**
   - Stir in soy sauce and hoisin sauce, and cook for another 2 minutes, ensuring everything is well-coated and heated through.

4. **Serve:**
   - Divide the stir-fry among four plates and serve hot.

4. Veggie-Packed Stuffed Bell Peppers

Serving Size: 4
Prep Time: 20 minutes
Cooking Time: 30 minutes

Nutrition Information (per serving):

- **Calories:** 320
- **Protein:** 12g
- **Carbohydrates:** 55g
- **Dietary Fiber:** 14g
- **Sugars:** 12g
- **Fat:** 8g
- **Saturated Fat:** 2g
- **Cholesterol:** 10mg

- **Sodium:** 450mg

Ingredients:

- 4 large bell peppers (any color), tops cut off and seeds removed
- 1 cup cooked brown rice
- 1 cup black beans, drained and rinsed
- 1 cup corn kernels (fresh or frozen)
- 1 cup diced tomatoes
- 1/2 cup shredded low-fat cheese (optional)
- 1 teaspoon cumin
- 1 teaspoon paprika
- Salt and pepper to taste
- Fresh cilantro for garnish

Directions:

1. **Preheat the Oven:** Preheat your oven to 375°F (190°C).
2. **Prepare the Filling:**
   - In a large bowl, combine the cooked brown rice, black beans, corn, diced tomatoes, cumin, paprika, salt, and pepper. Mix well to ensure all ingredients are evenly distributed.
3. **Stuff the Peppers:**
   - Spoon the filling into each bell pepper, packing it in tightly. Arrange the stuffed peppers upright in a baking dish.
4. **Bake:**

- Cover the baking dish with aluminum foil and bake in the preheated oven for 25 minutes.
- Remove the foil, sprinkle the tops with shredded low-fat cheese (if using), and bake for an additional 5 minutes, or until the cheese is melted and bubbly.

5. **Serve:**
- Garnish the stuffed bell peppers with fresh cilantro and serve hot. Enjoy as a standalone dish or pair with a side salad for a complete meal.

5. Zucchini Noodles with Pesto and Grilled Shrimp

Serving Size

This recipe serves 4.

Prep Time

15 minutes

Cooking Time

10 minutes

Nutrition Information (per serving)

- Calories: 240
- Protein: 20g
- Carbohydrates: 8g
- Dietary Fiber: 3g
- Sugars: 4g
- Fat: 14g
- Saturated Fat: 2g
- Sodium: 400mg

Ingredients

- 4 medium zucchinis, spiralized
- 1 lb large shrimp, peeled and deveined
- 2 tbsp olive oil
- 1/2 cup basil pesto (store-bought or homemade)
- 1/4 cup grated Parmesan cheese
- Juice of 1 lemon
- Salt and pepper to taste

Directions

1. **Prepare the Shrimp:**
   - Toss the shrimp with 1 tablespoon of olive oil, lemon juice, salt, and pepper.

- o Preheat the grill to medium-high heat. Grill the shrimp for 2-3 minutes on each side, until pink and cooked through. Remove from the grill and set aside.

2. **Cook the Zucchini Noodles:**
   - o In a large skillet, heat the remaining tablespoon of olive oil over medium heat.
   - o Add the spiralized zucchini to the skillet and sauté for 2-3 minutes until tender but still slightly crisp. Avoid overcooking as zucchini noodles can become watery.

3. **Combine and Serve:**
   - o Remove the skillet from heat and stir in the basil pesto, ensuring the zucchini noodles are well coated.
   - o Divide the zucchini noodles among four plates. Top each plate with the grilled shrimp.
   - o Sprinkle with grated Parmesan cheese for an added touch of flavor.

4. **Garnish:**
   - o Optionally, garnish with additional lemon juice or fresh basil leaves for extra freshness.

Tips for Success

- **Zucchini Noodles:** If you don't have a spiralizer, you can use a julienne peeler or buy pre-spiralized zucchini from the store.
- **Pesto:** For a homemade touch, you can make your own pesto using fresh basil, garlic, pine nuts, Parmesan cheese, and olive oil.
- **Shrimp:** Make sure the shrimp are fully thawed and patted dry before grilling to ensure even cooking and a nice sear.

6. Quinoa and Black Bean Stuffed Sweet Potatoes

Serving Size

This recipe serves 4.

Prep Time

20 minutes

Cooking Time

40 minutes

Nutrition Information (per serving)

- Calories: 350
- Protein: 10g
- Carbohydrates: 60g
- Dietary Fiber: 10g
- Sugars: 12g
- Fat: 6g
- Saturated Fat: 1g
- Sodium: 300mg
- Potassium: 950mg

Ingredients

- 4 medium sweet potatoes
- 1 cup cooked quinoa
- 1 cup black beans, drained and rinsed
- 1/2 cup corn kernels
- 1/2 cup diced tomatoes
- 1/4 cup chopped green onions
- 1 tsp chili powder
- 1 tsp cumin
- Salt and pepper to taste
- 1/4 cup Greek yogurt
- Fresh cilantro for garnish

Directions

1. **Preheat Oven:** Preheat your oven to 400°F (200°C).
2. **Bake Sweet Potatoes:** Pierce the sweet potatoes several times with a fork. Place them on a baking sheet and bake in the preheated oven for about 40

minutes, or until they are tender when pierced with a fork.

3. **Prepare Quinoa Filling:** While the sweet potatoes are baking, prepare the filling. In a large bowl, combine the cooked quinoa, black beans, corn, diced tomatoes, and chopped green onions. Season the mixture with chili powder, cumin, salt, and pepper. Mix well to ensure all ingredients are evenly distributed.

4. **Stuff Sweet Potatoes:** Once the sweet potatoes are done baking, remove them from the oven and let them cool slightly. Carefully slice each sweet potato open lengthwise and scoop out some of the flesh to create space for the filling. Spoon the quinoa and black bean mixture into each sweet potato.

5. **Add Toppings:** Top each stuffed sweet potato with a dollop of Greek yogurt and garnish with fresh cilantro for a burst of flavor and a touch of freshness.

6. **Serve:** Serve the stuffed sweet potatoes warm, and enjoy a nutritious and satisfying meal that's perfect for weight loss and packed with wholesome ingredients.

CONCLUSION

Congratulations on completing "Superb Weight Loss Cookbook for Beginners 2024"! You've taken a significant step towards transforming your health and well-being through delicious, nutritious meals. As you close this book, remember that healthy eating is a lifelong journey—one that is as rewarding as it is fulfilling.

Throughout these pages, you've discovered the power of wholesome ingredients, learned how to create balanced meals that support your weight loss goals, and gained valuable insights into building sustainable eating habits. Whether you're just starting out on your journey or looking to maintain your progress, the recipes and guidance provided here will continue to be your trusted companion.

Remember, healthy eating is not about perfection—it's about progress. Embrace the small victories and celebrate every step forward. Listen to your body, honor your cravings mindfully, and savor each meal as a nourishing gift to yourself.

As you move forward, continue to explore new flavors, experiment with different ingredients, and find joy in the process of cooking and eating well. Stay connected with your health goals and make adjustments as needed to ensure they align with your unique lifestyle and preferences.

Lastly, share your newfound knowledge and recipes with others. Spread the joy of healthy eating within your community and inspire those around you to embark on their own journey towards better health.

Thank you for choosing "Superb Weight Loss Cookbook for Beginners 2024." May your culinary adventures continue to bring you joy, vitality, and lasting health.

Warmest wishes,

Mary M. Vanish

Made in the USA
Columbia, SC
06 December 2024

48569844R00067